To enhance iron absorption, it is beneficial to pair iron-rich foods with vitamin C. For instance, enjoying a spinach salad with orange slices can provide this vital combination.

Calcium: Building Blocks for Bones

Calcium is crucial for the development of the baby's bones, teeth, muscles, and nerves. It also helps prevent the mother from losing bone density during pregnancy.

The recommended daily intake for pregnant women is around 1,000 milligrams. Good sources of calcium include:

- Dairy products like milk, cheese, and yogurt

- Fortified plant-based alternatives

- Leafy greens such as broccoli and kale

Ensuring adequate calcium intake can support both the mother's and baby's skeletal health.

Protein: The Building Block of Life

Protein plays a vital role in foetal tissue growth and placenta formation. During pregnancy, the protein needs of a woman rise significantly.

A daily goal of about 70 grams of protein is recommended. Sources include:

- Lean meats and poultry

- Fish such as salmon and tuna.

- Eggs, beans, nuts, and seeds

Diversifying protein sources not only meets these needs but also fulfills additional nutritional requirements.

Vitamin D and Iodine: Micronutrients that Matter

Vitamin D is essential for bone health and helps in calcium absorption. Pregnant women should aim for about 600 IU of vitamin

D daily. This can be obtained through sunlight, fortified foods, and fatty fish like salmon.

Iodine, essential for brain and thyroid development, has an intake goal of 220 micrograms per day for pregnant women. Good sources include:

- Iodized salt

- Dairy products

- Seafood

Adequate iodine levels are crucial for the baby's neurological development.

Choline and Omega-3 Fatty Acids: Brain Development Allies

Choline is vital for brain development and cell membrane construction. Pregnant women should aim for around 450 milligrams of choline daily, found in:

- Eggs

- Lean meats

- Beans

Omega-3 fatty acids are equally important, contributing to foetal brain and eye development. Pregnant women should target 200 to 300 milligrams of DHA and EPA daily, available in:

- Fatty fish like salmon

- Walnuts and chia seeds

Hydration and Caloric Intake: Balancing the Equation

Hydration is often overlooked but remains a cornerstone of pregnancy health. Sufficient fluids help maintain amniotic fluid levels, support kidney function, and alleviate discomforts such as swelling.

Pregnancy Wellness: Essential Nutrition and Diet Secrets

Chapter 1: Introduction to Pregnancy and Nutrition

Pregnancy is a remarkable and transformative period in a woman's life. It involves not only the growth of a new life but also significant changes to the mother's body. Consequently, good nutrition is paramount during these nine months as it plays a crucial role in the health and development of both mother and baby. This chapter will provide an overview of why nutrition matters so much during pregnancy, highlight the key dietary considerations, and set the stage for the more detailed discussions in later chapters.

- **Understanding Nutritional Needs:** Pregnancy increases the body's demand for certain nutrients. Understanding these needs is the first step to ensuring a healthy pregnancy.

- **The Impact on Baby's Development:** Your diet directly impacts your baby's growth and development, influencing everything from birth weight to cognitive development.

- **Your Changing Body:** Pregnancy causes changes in metabolism and dietary requirements, making personalized nutrition plans essential.

Understanding Nutritional Needs

Pregnancy marks a remarkable chapter in a woman's life. As her body adapts to support a growing baby, it needs a precise blend of nutrients for both health and development. Knowing what to eat during this time is crucial. The right nutrition not only supports the mother's well-being but also sets a strong foundation for the baby's growth. By exploring the essential nutrients needed at various stages of pregnancy, new mums can effectively nourish themselves and their little ones.

The Importance of Nutritional Needs in Pregnancy

Pregnancy brings about substantial changes in the body, increasing the demand for specific vitamins and minerals. These nutrients are vital for foetal growth and maternal health, helping reduce the chances of complications such as gestational diabetes and preterm labour. A balanced diet rich in essential nutrients can help alleviate common pregnancy challenges like fatigue and nausea, providing not only energy but also overall wellness.

Folic Acid: The Essential Vitamin

Folic acid is perhaps the most important nutrient for pregnant women. This B vitamin aids in DNA synthesis and cell division, and it significantly lowers the risk of neural tube defects in newborns. Pregnant women are advised to consume 600 micrograms of folic acid daily through food and prenatal vitamins.

Sources of folic acid include:

- Leafy greens like spinach and kale

- Legumes such as lentils and chickpeas

- Fortified cereals and grains

Incorporating these foods into daily meals can support the foetal brain and spinal cord development, which is critical especially in the early stages of pregnancy.

Iron: Fighting Fatigue

Iron is essential for producing haemoglobin, which carries oxygen to both mother and baby. As blood volume increases during pregnancy, so does the need for iron. Insufficient iron can lead to anaemia, causing fatigue and weakness.

Pregnant women should aim for about 27 milligrams of iron each day. Excellent sources include:

- Lean meats like chicken and beef

- Beans and lentils

- Spinach and fortified cereals

Caloric needs also increase, particularly in the second and third trimesters, where an additional 300 calories per day is recommended. Focus should be on nutrient-rich foods rather than empty calories to promote healthy gains for both mother and baby.

Trimester-Specific Needs: Tailoring Nutrition Throughout Pregnancy

Nutritional requirements evolve throughout pregnancy.

- **First trimester:** Focus on folic acid and other essential vitamins for foetal development.

- **Second trimester:** Increased caloric and protein intake as the baby grows rapidly.

- **Third trimester:** Emphasize calcium, iron, and hydration in preparation for labour and breastfeeding.

Understanding these trimester-specific needs enables new mums to make informed dietary choices that reflect their body's changing requirements.

Being aware of nutritional needs during pregnancy goes beyond simply eating for two. It entails recognizing what nutrients are vital for both mother and baby. By emphasizing a balanced diet rich in folic acid, iron, calcium, protein, vitamin D, choline, and omega-3 fatty acids, new mums can support a healthy pregnancy and promote their children's future wellness.

Consulting a healthcare professional or registered dietitian can provide customized guidance tailored to individual needs. With a thoughtful approach to nutrition, pregnancy can be a time of strength and nourishment, as mothers prepare to bring their little ones into the world.

With informed food choices, hydration, and a clear understanding of trimester-specific needs, navigating pregnancy nutrition can be both fulfilling and enriching.

When it comes to pregnancy, many expectant mothers focus on essential factors such as prenatal vitamins and baby gear. However, the impact of a mother's diet on her baby's development is often understated. Research increasingly indicates that maternal nutrition affects everything from birth weight to cognitive abilities and long-term health. This post examines the significant connection between a mother's dietary choices and her baby's developmental milestones.

The Importance of Birth Weight

Birth weight is a vital indicator of a newborn's health. Babies with low birth weight (less than 5.5 pounds) face a higher risk of developing difficulties such as learning delays and motor skill challenges. For instance, studies reveal that about 20% of low-birth-weight infants may have developmental impairments that persist into childhood.

Maternal nutrition plays a crucial role in determining birth weight. A study published in the *American Journal of Clinical Nutrition* found that women who consumed a diet rich in fruits, vegetables, and whole grains had infants with birth weights that were, on average, 4 ounces heavier than those with less nutritious diets. Key nutrients like protein, iron, and omega-3 fatty acids not only facilitate the growth of foetal organs but also support brain development, which is crucial for the infant's overall health.

Cognitive Development: The Role of Nutrition

Cognitive development in infants starts in the womb and continues throughout early childhood. A mother's diet has profound effects on brain development, influencing indicators such as IQ scores, brain volume, and cognitive abilities. Nutrients like folic acid, found in leafy greens and fortified cereals, are essential for preventing neural tube defects and supporting healthy brain formation.

Research shows that infants whose mothers included omega-3 fatty acids, commonly found in fish, in their diet had brain development advantages. For example, a study indicated that children whose mothers consumed adequate levels of omega-3s scored an average of 5 points higher on IQ tests than those whose diets were lacking in these vital fats.

Maternal Influences: Socioeconomic Factors and Lifestyle

Maternal nutrition should be viewed alongside other factors like socioeconomic status and lifestyle choices. Studies indicate that maternal smoking, inadequate prenatal care, and high stress levels can impede foetal growth and contribute to low birth weight. These elements not only negatively affect physical health but also correlate with cognitive outcomes. For example, children born to mothers who smoked during pregnancy are at a 30% higher risk of developmental delays.

On the other side, good perinatal care and balanced nutrition can help counter some negative influences. Mothers from higher socioeconomic backgrounds often have better access to nutritious food and prenatal services. This access can lead to healthier birth outcomes and better cognitive development. For example, infants born to mothers in this demographic are typically 1 pound heavier at birth on average.

The Long-Term Health Effects of Nutritional Choices

Nutrition impacts not just a baby's immediate health but their long-term health as well. Research highlights that maternal diet during pregnancy can increase the risk of chronic conditions later in life. Children whose mothers consumed diets high in processed foods during pregnancy may face a 25% higher risk of developing obesity and diabetes as they grow older.

By choosing nutrient-dense foods, mothers can help their children avoid certain health risks. Adequate nutrition during pregnancy lays a strong foundation for not just birth weight and cognitive development, but also overall health throughout the child's life.

Essential Nutrients for Expecting Mothers

To promote better birth outcomes and cognitive development, expectant mothers should focus on incorporating specific nutrients into their diets. Key nutrients include:

- **Folic Acid**: Necessary for reducing the risk of neural tube defects. Women are advised to begin supplementation with folic acid at least one month before conception.

- **Iron**: Important for maintaining healthy blood flow and energy. Rich sources of iron include lean meats, beans, and fortified cereals.

- **Omega-3 Fatty Acids**: Essential for developing brain function. Excellent sources include fatty fish, walnuts, and flaxseeds.

- **Calcium and Vitamin D**: Crucial for bone health and development. These nutrients can be sourced from dairy products, leafy greens, and sun exposure.

- **Protein**: Important for foetal tissue and organ growth. Lean meats, eggs, beans, and dairy are all excellent sources.

Expectant mothers should strive for a balanced diet featuring these nutrients to nurture their babies' health effectively.

Practical Tips for Maintaining a Balanced Diet

Maintaining a nutritious diet during pregnancy is achievable with a few simple strategies:

1. **Plan Meals**: Outline a weekly menu centred around nutrient-rich foods. This will make it easier to shop and prepare meals.

2. **Smart Snacking**: Choose healthy snacks like fruits, nuts, or yogurt, steering clear of sugary options.

3. **Hydrate**: Stay hydrated by drinking plenty of water throughout the day. Proper hydration supports overall bodily functions.

4. **Consult Professionals**: Regular consultations with healthcare providers can help ensure dietary needs are being met effectively.

5. **Stay Informed**: Understanding proper food choices can empower mothers to make better decisions. Familiarizing oneself with nutrition labels can help as well.

The connection between a mother's diet and her baby's development is significant and far-reaching. Maternal choices influence birth weight, cognitive development, and even long-term health. By prioritizing nutrition, expectant mothers can give their children a solid foundation for a healthy life. Understanding this link equips new mothers with the tools they need to support their child's health during critical developmental years and beyond. Remember, "You are what you eat," is especially true during pregnancy's transformative journey.

Your Changing Body

Pregnancy is an incredible journey, transforming a woman's body to nurture new life. These transformations bring significant changes, particularly to metabolism and dietary needs. Recognizing these adjustments is essential for expectant mothers to ensure their own well-being and that of their developing baby. This post will explore how pregnancy impacts metabolism and why personalized nutrition plans are crucial for new mums.

The Impact of Pregnancy on Metabolism

The hormonal shifts during pregnancy noticeably affect metabolism. From conception onward, the body gears up to support the growth of the foetus.

A key change is the rise in basal metabolic rate (BMR), which indicates the calories needed to sustain essential bodily functions at rest. Research shows that a woman's BMR can increase by about 10 to 15 percent during the first trimester alone. This increase means that expectant mums should expect to consume more calories, approximately an additional 300 to 500 calories a day, particularly in the second and third trimesters to support foetal development and breast milk production.

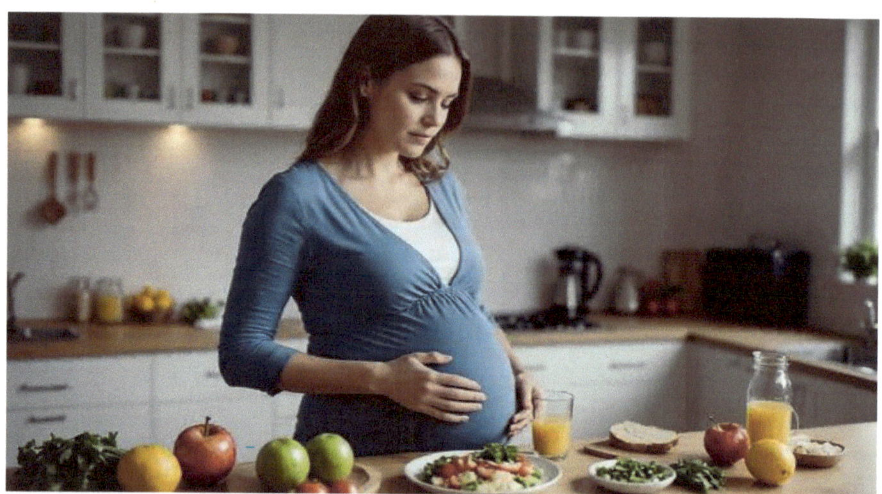

Further, hormonal changes can cause increased insulin resistance. This is a natural process that ensures that enough glucose is available for foetal nourishment. However, it may also lead to conditions like gestational diabetes, emphasizing the need for frequent monitoring and tailored dietary strategies.

Understanding Dietary Requirements

As the body adapts to support the growing foetus, the dietary requirements of pregnant women become crucial. Attention to both macronutrients and micronutrients is necessary to fuel both the mother and the developing baby.

Macronutrients: Carbohydrates, Proteins, and Fats

- **Carbohydrates**: Pregnant women benefit from increased carbohydrate intake to maintain energy levels, especially in the second and third trimesters. A diet rich in whole grains, fruits, and vegetables can provide essential fiber and nutrients. A study found that women who consumed adequate whole grains had a 30% lower risk of gestational diabetes.

- **Protein**: Protein needs become particularly significant, with recommendations set at around 75 to 100 grams per day depending on the trimester. High-protein foods, such as lean meats, legumes, and dairy, support foetal growth and help maintain maternal muscle health.

- **Fats**: Healthy fats are vital for foetal brain development. Incorporating omega-3 rich foods like salmon or flaxseeds can contribute to optimal cognitive outcomes for the baby.

Micronutrients: The Building Blocks for Health

Micronutrients, including essential vitamins and minerals, are fundamental during pregnancy. Key nutrients to prioritize include:

- **Folic Acid**: Crucial for preventing neural tube defects, women are advised to start folic acid supplements even before conception. A potent source is leafy greens and fortified cereals.

- **Iron**: Blood volume increases during pregnancy, raising iron needs to prevent anaemia. Pregnant women should consume approximately 27 mg of iron daily. Foods high in iron, such as lean red meat, legumes, and fortified cereals, should be included regularly.

- **Calcium**: Essential for bone health, pregnant women need around 1,000 mg of calcium daily. Good sources include dairy products, leafy greens, and fortified plant-based milks.

Hydration is also critical, as increased blood volume and nutrient transportation require adequate fluid intake.

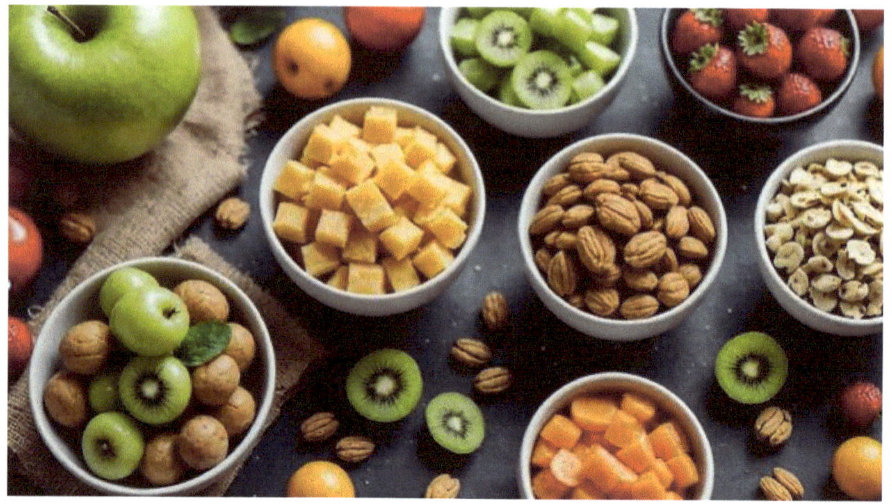

Tailoring a Personalized Nutrition Plan

Given the metabolic shifts and distinct dietary requirements, creating personalized nutrition plans is vital for pregnant women. Understanding individual needs—based on factors like pre-pregnancy weight, existing health conditions, and daily activity—can enhance health outcomes.

Nutritional Assessment

Conducting a thorough nutritional assessment early in pregnancy can be beneficial. This assessment may include:

- **Evaluating dietary habits**: Keeping a food diary to identify nutritional gaps ensures that mothers make informed food choices.

- **Assessing lifestyle factors**: Considering physical activity, socio-economic status, and food access can help form realistic dietary recommendations.

- **Monitoring health conditions**: For mothers with conditions like diabetes, specialized nutrition plans can help manage insulin resistance and support a healthy pregnancy.

Trimester-Specific Needs

Acknowledging that nutritional requirements change across trimesters allows for more effective personalization. Here are some examples:

- **First Trimester**: Focus on folic acid, hydration, and managing nausea with nutrient-dense snacks, such as whole-grain toast or yogurt with fruit.

- **Second Trimester**: Concentrate on increased protein and calcium intake, with recommended foods like Greek yogurt, lean meats, and fortified drinks.

- **Third Trimester**: Heightened caloric intake—roughly 300 to 500 additional calories—is needed to support significant foetal growth and maternal energy demands.

Transitioning from generic dietary advice to a personalized plan can prevent excessive weight gain and reduce risks associated with gestational diabetes.

Embracing the Journey of Nutrition

Navigating dietary requirements during pregnancy presents unique challenges. As metabolism changes, adhering to a personalized nutrition plan is vital for both the health of the mother and the baby. By prioritizing essential macronutrients and micronutrients and tailoring dietary plans to individual needs, new mums can thrive throughout their pregnancy journey.

Consultation with healthcare professionals can provide invaluable guidance in developing a nutrition plan that caters to specific needs. By taking proactive steps in nutrition today, new mothers can set the stage for a healthier future for themselves and their children.

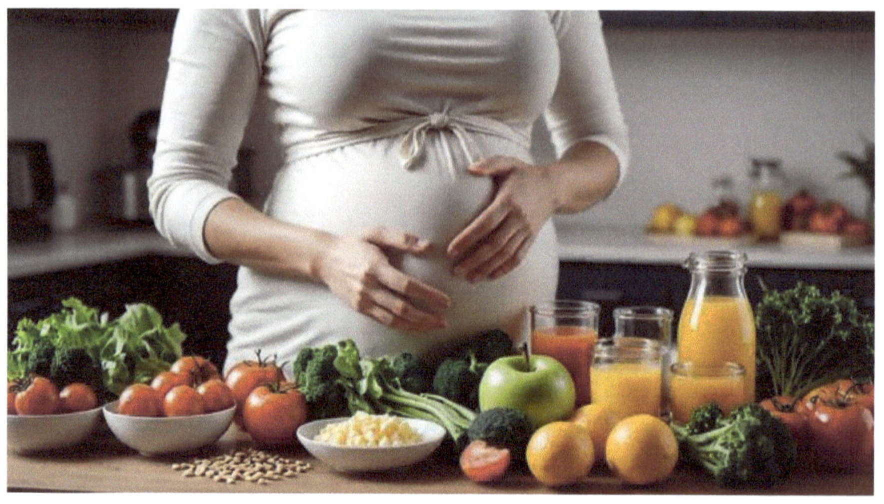

Chapter 2: Essential Nutrients for a Healthy Pregnancy

Folic Acid

Folic acid is critical in the early stages of pregnancy and plays a vital role in preventing neural tube defects. Learn about:

- **Recommended intake**

- **Sources like leafy greens, legumes, and fortified cereals**

- **Timing and supplementation**

Folic acid, a crucial B-vitamin, is essential during pregnancy, especially in the early stages when significant bodily changes occur. Its importance is highlighted by its role in preventing neural tube defects (NTDs), which can lead to serious conditions like spina bifida and anencephaly. In this post, we will explore the recommended intake, dietary sources, and effective strategies for supplementation, giving expectant mothers the information they need to protect their babies' health.

Recommended Intake of Folic Acid

For women in the periconceptional period, which spans from one to three months before conception until the end of the first trimester, the recommended intake of folic acid ranges from **400 to 800 micrograms (mcg) per day**. This increase is vital because adequate folate levels are essential for DNA and RNA synthesis, as well as the development of foetal tissues.

Interestingly, research shows that **50% of all pregnancies are unplanned**. This statistic underscores the importance of folic acid supplementation for all women of reproductive age, not just those planning to become pregnant. By maintaining sufficient folic acid levels before pregnancy, women can significantly reduce the risk of NTDs.

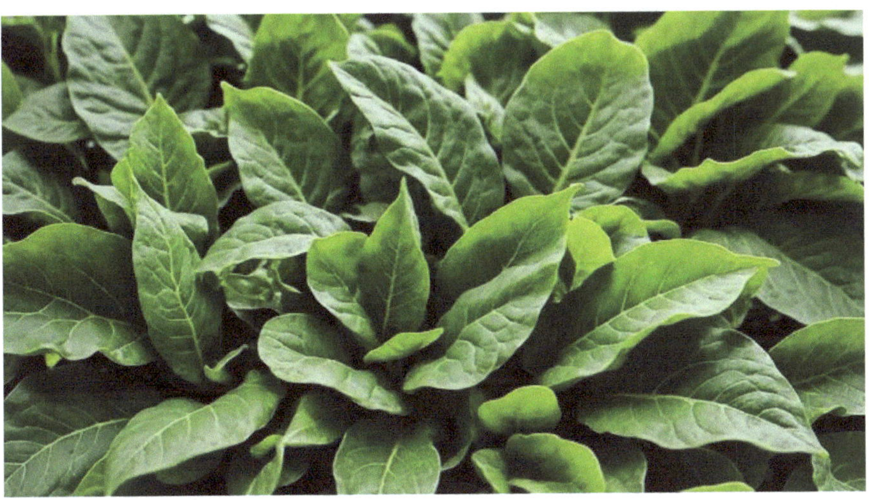

Dietary Sources of Folic Acid

Incorporating a variety of folic acid-rich foods into your diet can help meet daily requirements while also being delicious.

Leafy Greens

Leafy greens like spinach, kale, and Swiss chard are among the best sources of folic acid. For instance, one cup of cooked spinach provides approximately **263 mcg of folate**, which is about **66% of the daily requirement**. Adding these greens to salads, smoothies, or soups can significantly boost folic acid intake.

Legumes

Legumes such as lentils, chickpeas, and beans are also excellent sources of folic acid. A single cup of cooked lentils contains about **358 mcg of folate**, which accounts for nearly **90%** of the daily recommended intake! These versatile foods can be included in various meals like dips, soups, and salads, making them easy to incorporate into daily diets.

Fortified Cereals

Many breakfast cereals are fortified with folic acid, providing an easy way to increase intake. For example, just one serving of fortified cereal can offer between **100 to 400 mcg** of folic acid. When selecting cereals, choose those low in sugar and high in fiber to maximize health benefits.

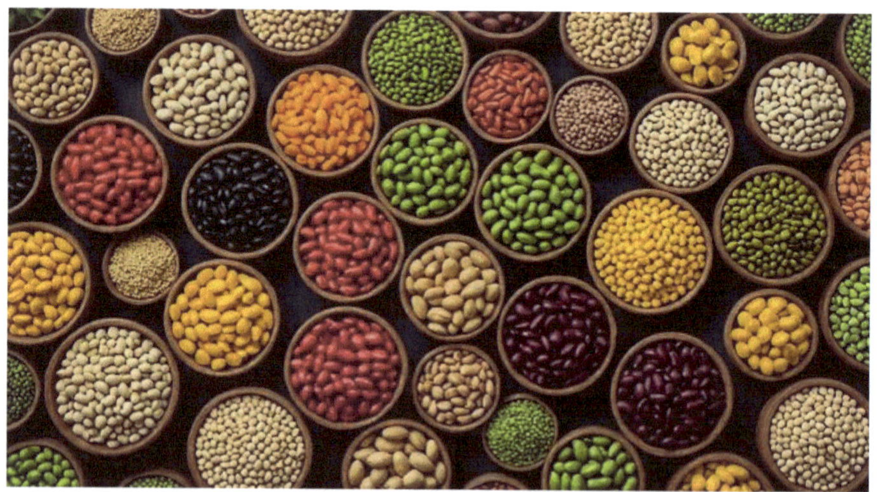

Timing and Supplementation

The right timing for folic acid intake is crucial in preventing neural tube defects. Research indicates that neural tube formation happens within the first few weeks of pregnancy, often before a woman even realizes she is pregnant. Therefore, starting supplementation as soon as you begin trying to conceive is key.

For those with a history of NTDs in previous pregnancies, higher doses of folic acid—up to **4,000 mcg**—may be recommended. Always consult a healthcare provider before starting any supplementation to determine the right dosage for your personal health needs.

Combining folic acid with other B vitamins, particularly vitamin B12, can enhance its effectiveness. Both vitamins play essential roles in processes like methylation and homocysteine metabolism, which may influence neural tube development.

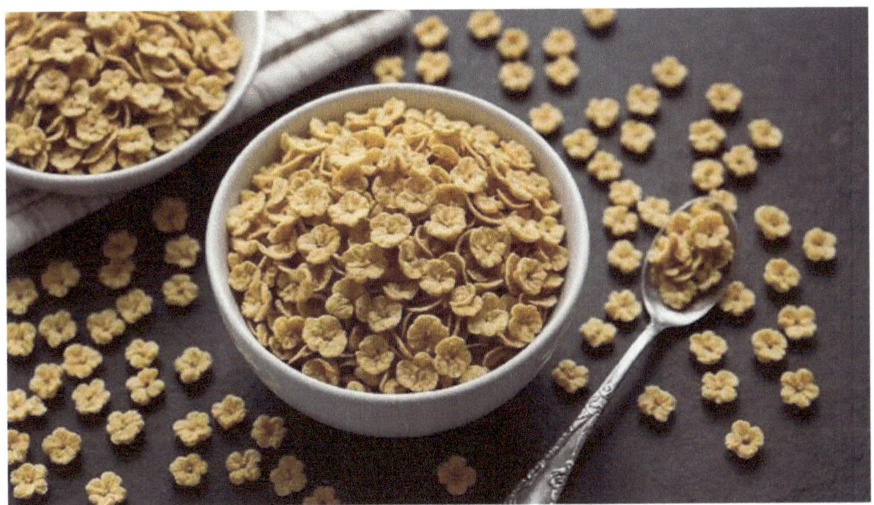

Exploring Folic Acid's Role in Cellular Functions

Folic acid is vital for several cellular processes, including DNA synthesis and repair, as well as the production of red and white blood cells. It also plays a significant role in methylation—when methyl groups are added to DNA, influencing genetic expression and health outcomes.

Understanding genetic factors, such as variations in the MTHFR gene, which affect folate metabolism can help develop personalized dietary strategies. Individuals with MTHFR polymorphisms may require higher levels of folate to achieve adequate status, emphasizing the need for tailored nutritional approaches during pregnancy.

Final Thoughts on Folic Acid in Pregnancy

Folic acid is fundamental to maternal health and vital for preventing neural tube defects during early pregnancy stages. With a recommended intake of **400 to 800 mcg per day**, dietary sources like leafy greens, legumes, and fortified cereals can greatly assist in meeting these needs.

By starting supplementation before pregnancy and understanding the importance of folic acid, particularly for women with a history of NTDs, expectant mothers can make informed choices. Incorporating these practices into daily life not only paves the way for a healthy pregnancy but also creates a nurturing environment for the growing baby.

Always consult with healthcare providers for personalized guidance to ensure the best outcomes as you embark on the journey of motherhood.

Iron

Iron supports the increased blood volume during pregnancy and prevents anaemia.

- **Daily requirements and food sources such as red meat, lentils, and spinach**

- **Tips to enhance iron absorption.**

Pregnancy brings many changes to a woman's body. These changes require careful attention to nutrition, especially in terms of iron intake. Iron is key for producing haemoglobin, which helps transport oxygen throughout the body. This blog post will explain the daily iron requirements for new moms, highlight iron-rich food sources, and provide practical tips to enhance iron absorption.

The Importance of Iron During Pregnancy

Iron is critical for several reasons during pregnancy. A woman's blood volume increases by about 50% during this time, meaning she needs more iron to support both her body and the developing baby. If iron levels drop too low, women may develop iron deficiency anaemia, which can lead to symptoms like fatigue and weakness. According to studies, approximately **15-25% of pregnant women experience some form of anaemia.** In severe cases, anaemia can result in complications, such as preterm delivery and low birth weight.

Ensuring sufficient iron intake supports not only the mother's health but also the baby's healthy development. New moms should be aware of their iron needs throughout pregnancy to avoid potential risks.

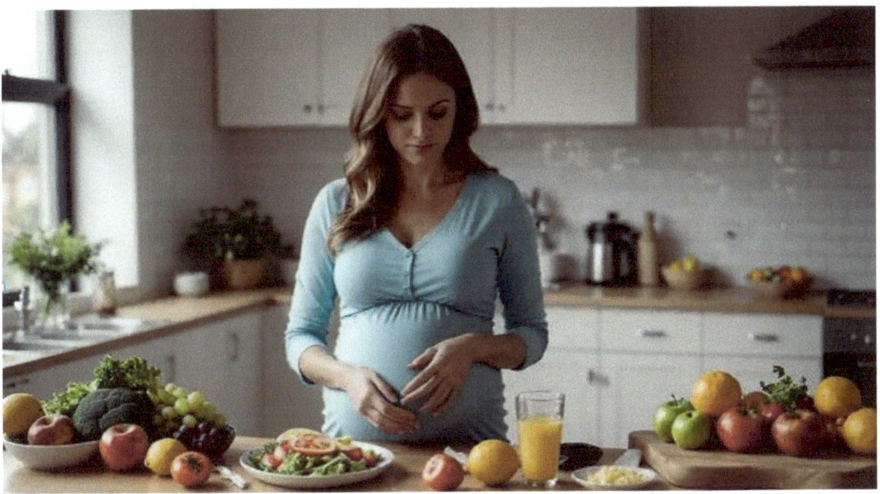

Daily Iron Requirements for New Moms

Daily iron requirements change based on individual health and the pregnancy stage. The recommended dietary allowance (RDA) is **27 mg of iron per day for pregnant women**, significantly higher than the average intake for non-pregnant women, which is around **18 mg**. For breastfeeding mothers, the requirement drops to approximately **9-10 mg per day**.

Monitoring iron intake is essential, especially in the second and third trimesters when the body's iron needs peak. Healthcare providers can help new moms assess their iron status and suggest dietary changes or supplements as needed.

Food Sources of Iron

It is crucial to include a variety of food sources in the diet to meet daily iron needs. Iron comes in two types: heme iron and non-heme iron.

Heme Iron

Heme iron, found in animal products, is more easily absorbed than non-heme iron. Foods rich in heme iron include:

- **Red Meat**: Beef is one of the best sources, providing about **2.1 mg of iron per 3-ounce serving**.

- **Poultry**: Chicken and turkey are excellent options, offering around **1.1 mg of iron per 3-ounce serving**.

- **Fish**: Especially shellfish like clams or oysters, which can contain up to **28 mg of iron per 3-ounce serving**.

Non-Heme Iron

Non-heme iron is found primarily in plant-based foods and is less readily absorbed but still important. It is available in:

- **Lentils**: One cup offers **6.6 mg of iron**, along with fiber and protein.

- **Spinach**: One cup cooked provides **6.4 mg of iron**, while also delivering essential vitamins.

- **Fortified Cereals**: Many breakfast cereals contain added iron, ranging from **10-45% of the daily value per serving**.

Incorporating these foods into daily meals can help meet iron intake recommendations during pregnancy.

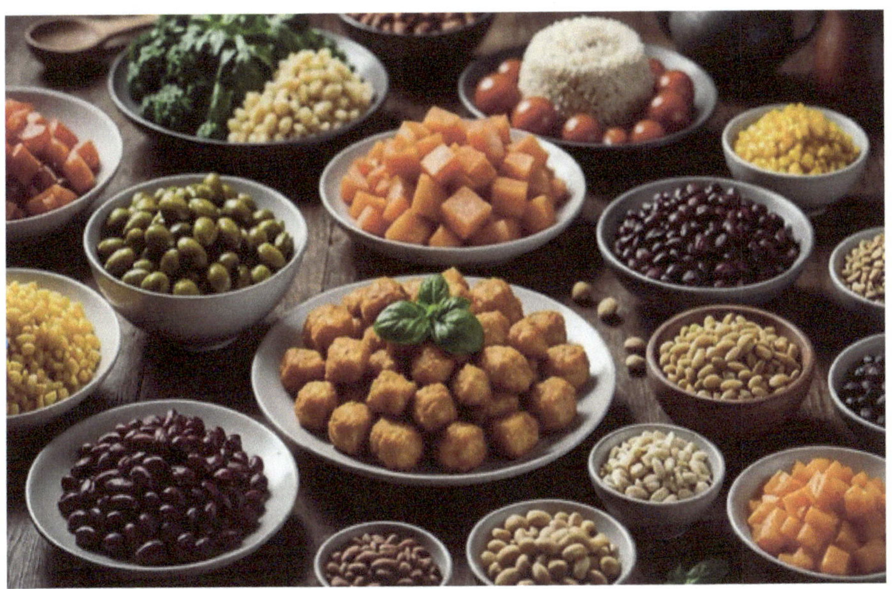

Tips to Enhance Iron Absorption

Eating iron-rich foods is important, but there are specific strategies to improve iron absorption. Here are some effective tips:

Pair Iron with Vitamin C

Consuming vitamin C alongside non-heme iron can significantly enhance absorption. For instance, pair a serving of lentils with a salad topped with bell peppers or have strawberries with fortified cereal. This simple combination can substantially increase your body's ability to take in iron from these foods.

Avoid Calcium and Tannins During Iron-Rich Meals

Certain substances can block iron absorption. Calcium, found in dairy products, competes with iron in the intestines. Similarly, tannins from tea and coffee can hinder absorption. To maximize iron intake, try to separate dairy products and these beverages from iron-rich meals by at least two hours.

Consider Cooking Methods

How you cook can also affect iron levels. Cooking in cast iron cookware can increase the iron content of foods, particularly acidic foods like tomato sauce. Using this method can provide a simple boost to your daily iron intake.

Supplements When Necessary

If dietary changes do not suffice, pregnant women should discuss iron supplements with their healthcare provider. Some women might be at risk for iron deficiency, making monitoring ferritin levels through blood tests essential for assessing their needs.

Final Thoughts on Iron for New Moms

Iron is a critical nutrient that greatly affects the health and well-being of new mothers during pregnancy. Striving to meet daily iron requirements through a mix of heme and non-heme sources is vital for preventing anaemia and supporting the increased blood volume essential during this life-changing period.

From enjoying red meat to integrating lentils and spinach into meals, there are plenty of tasty options to choose from. By adopting effective absorption strategies and consulting healthcare professionals about potential supplementation, mothers can actively support their iron levels.

Understanding the importance of iron and making mindful dietary choices will help new moms ensure a healthy pregnancy and a thriving future.

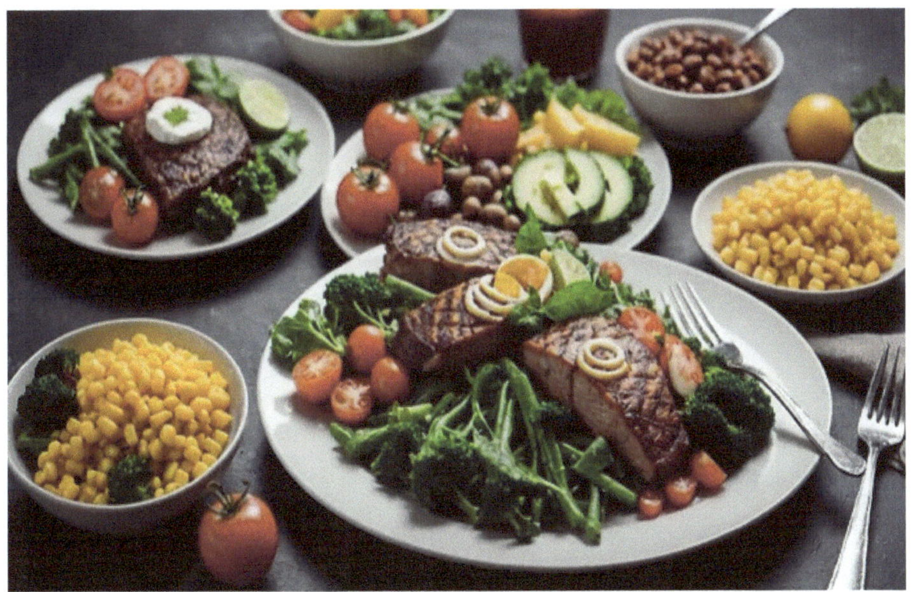

Calcium

Calcium is essential for developing your baby's bones and teeth.

Calcium plays a crucial role during pregnancy, especially in developing your baby's bones and teeth. Getting enough calcium is essential for both foetal growth and the mother's health. As your body undergoes various changes, knowing the right calcium amounts, sources, and potential health implications can help ensure a healthy pregnancy.

Why Calcium is Crucial During Pregnancy

Calcium is a key mineral that supports strong bone and teeth formation in your developing baby. As pregnancy progresses, your baby's skeletal system develops quickly, with calcium acting as a fundamental building block. According to studies, babies absorb calcium from their mothers, making adequate intake during pregnancy vital.

Additionally, sufficient calcium levels can help prevent complications for mothers, such as osteoporosis and high blood pressure disorders like preeclampsia. Research shows that women with higher calcium intake during pregnancy have up to a 40% lower risk of developing preeclampsia. A strong maternal bone density supports not only pregnancy but overall motherhood.

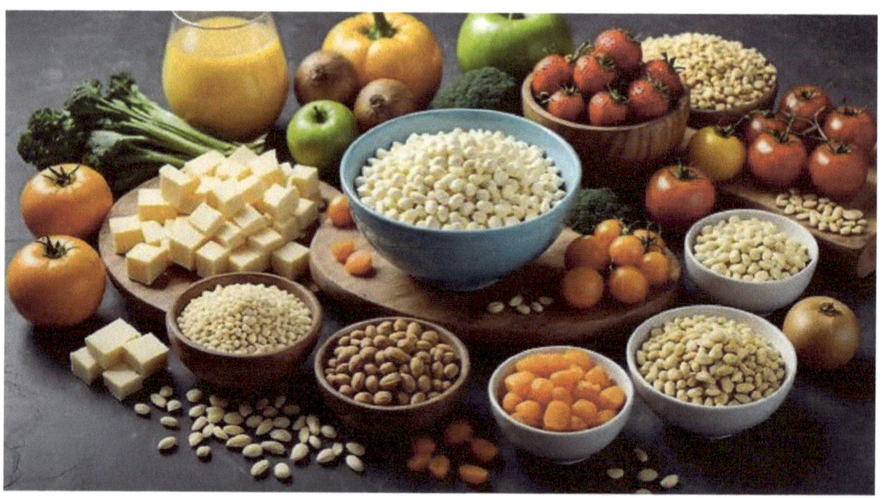

Recommended Calcium Intake for Pregnant Women

Pregnant women should aim for a daily intake of about **1,000 mg** of calcium. For teens aged 14 to 18, this requirement increases to **1,300 mg** per day as their bodies are still growing. Research indicates that only one in three pregnant women meet the recommended calcium intake, which underscores the importance of dietary vigilance.

During pregnancy, your body becomes more efficient at absorbing calcium, but the growing foetus's needs increase the importance of monitoring calcium levels. Incorporating calcium-rich foods into your daily diet can help meet these needs effectively.

Calcium-Rich Foods

There are many delicious options to help meet your calcium needs. For example:

Dairy Products

Dairy products are often the go-to choices when thinking about calcium. One cup of whole milk contains about **300 mg** of calcium, while a 6-ounce serving of yogurt can contain around **400 mg**.

Cheese can also be calcium-rich; for instance, one ounce of cheddar cheese provides approximately **200 mg** of calcium.

Fortified Alternatives

For those who might be lactose intolerant or prefer non-dairy options, many fortified alternatives are available. Popular choices include almond, soy, and oat milks, which can contain about **300 mg** of calcium per cup. Always check product labels to ensure you are getting enough calcium for your needs.

Leafy Greens

Leafy green vegetables are not just for salads; they are also packed with calcium. For example, one cup of cooked collard greens offers around **266 mg** of calcium, while kale provides about **94 mg** per cup. Including these in your meals can enhance your calcium intake significantly.

Fish

Certain fish, particularly sardines and canned salmon with bones, are excellent sources of calcium. A **3-ounce** serving of sardines contains about **325 mg** of calcium, making this a great option for seafood lovers.

Tofu

Tofu is another great way to boost calcium intake, especially if it is prepared with calcium sulphate. A half-cup serving can provide approximately **253 mg** of calcium, making it an excellent protein source for vegetarians and vegans.

Importance of Vitamin D

In addition to calcium, vitamin D is crucial for absorption. It helps in the mineralization of bones and teeth, ensuring that the calcium you take in effectively contributes to your baby's development. You can obtain vitamin D from sunlight, fortified foods, and supplements. Pregnant women should consult their healthcare provider to determine if they need additional vitamin D, especially if sunlight exposure is limited.

Calcium Supplements

If you struggle to meet your calcium amounts through food alone, supplements may be beneficial. They can effectively increase calcium levels during pregnancy. However, it is important to consult a healthcare provider before starting any supplements. Excessive calcium intake can lead to complications, including a higher risk of kidney stones.

Potential Risks of Low Calcium Intake

Low calcium intake during pregnancy can have serious consequences. Insufficient calcium may lead to decreased maternal bone density, raising the risk of osteoporosis. This is particularly concerning as women age. Additionally, low calcium can increase the likelihood of pregnancy complications like preeclampsia, which affects about **5-8%** of pregnancies globally.

For the developing baby, inadequate calcium can lead to poor bone formation and an elevated risk of fractures after birth. Ensuring that calcium needs are met through diet and supplements is essential for both mother and baby.

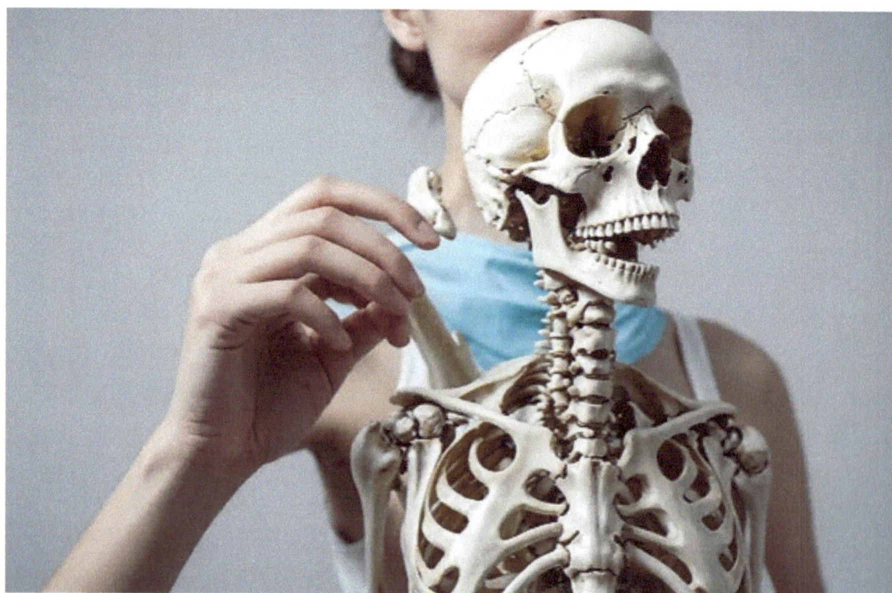

Prioritizing Calcium in Your Diet

Calcium's role in foetal growth and maternal health during pregnancy cannot be overstated. By focusing on a balanced intake of dairy products, fortified alternatives, greens, and fish, mothers can promote their baby's bone development and support their overall health.

Regular discussions with healthcare providers can also help establish a personalized nutritional strategy that considers both calcium needs and individual dietary habits. By prioritizing calcium intake, mothers can nurture healthy bones in their babies and lay a solid foundation for their family's long-term health.

Basically, adding calcium to your pregnancy diet is about more than preventing deficiencies; it sets the stage for your baby's healthy future. With mindful nutrition practices, you can make this beautiful journey of pregnancy even more rewarding.

Protein

Protein is the building block of life, crucial for your baby's growth and development.

- **Guidelines for protein intake**

- **High-quality protein sources like lean meats, tofu, and beans**

As a new mum, the journey of ensuring your baby's healthy growth can be both exciting and challenging. One crucial element of your baby's nutrition is protein. Often called the building block of life, protein is essential for your baby's muscle development, tissue growth, and overall well-being. This guide will equip you with valuable information on protein intake guidelines, high-quality protein sources, and practical ways to meet your baby's protein needs.

Understanding Protein Requirements

Your baby's protein needs change significantly, especially in the first year. Infants need sufficient protein for growth and health.

Protein is crucial for developing muscles, skin, enzymes, and hormones.

For newborns and infants, the recommended dietary allowance (RDA) generally falls between **1.5 to 2.2 grams of protein per kilogram of body weight**. For example, a 10-kilogram (22-pound) infant would need approximately **15 to 22 grams of protein each day**. It is wise to consult a paediatrician to get tailored guidelines based on your baby's health and growth patterns.

Additionally, protein requirements during pregnancy vary. The first and second trimesters typically need less protein compared to the third trimester, where the need may increase by up to 50% due to rapid foetal growth. This balance supports both maternal health and foetal development.

High-Quality Protein Sources

When choosing protein sources for your baby, it is essential to select high-quality proteins that include all the essential amino acids. Complete proteins can be derived from both animal and plant-based sources. Here are some top recommendations:

Lean Meats

Lean meats, such as chicken, turkey, and lean beef, are excellent protein sources. They not only provide significant protein but also essential vitamins and minerals that boost your baby's development.

Once your baby begins eating solids, consider introducing finely chopped, well-cooked meats. For example, **3 ounces of cooked chicken contains about 25 grams of protein**, making it a substantial addition to your baby's meals.

Fish and Poultry

Fish is another excellent protein source rich in omega-3 fatty acids, which are vital for brain development. Opt for safer options like salmon or trout, which are less likely to contain harmful levels of mercury.

For instance, **3 ounces of cooked salmon offers roughly 22 grams of protein** and supports cognitive health. Poultry, like chicken, is also highly nutritious and easy to digest.

Eggs and Dairy Products

Eggs are a fantastic protein source and can be introduced to your baby after six months. A large egg contains about **6 grams of protein**. Serving them well-cooked ensures safety and digestibility.

Dairy products, such as yogurt and cheese, provide good protein and calcium. For infants, **whole milk yogurt** is recommended, as it promotes healthy growth with necessary calories.

Legumes, Tofu, and Beans

Plant-based proteins are becoming popular and offer a diverse option for your baby. Legumes like lentils and chickpeas are excellent choices. For example, **1 cup of cooked lentils contains around 18 grams of protein** along with fiber, which promotes healthy digestion.

Tofu can also be a great addition. It is versatile and easy to mash, making it suitable for various dishes. Ensure that plant-based foods complement your baby's overall diet for balanced nutrition.

Nuts and Seeds

For babies over one year, finely ground nuts and seeds can enhance protein and healthy fat intake. For example, **2 tablespoons of almond butter provide about 7 grams of protein**. These can be added to smoothies or oatmeal.

However, whole nuts pose a choking risk, so they should be avoided for younger babies. Always consult your healthcare provider before introducing new foods to determine age-appropriate options.

Key Takeaways for New Mums

Protein is crucial for your baby's growth and development. By understanding protein requirements and selecting the best sources, you can confidently provide optimal nutrition for your little one.

Incorporating high-quality proteins such as lean meats, fish, poultry, eggs, dairy products, legumes, tofu, beans, nuts, and seeds will greatly benefit your baby's muscle and tissue growth, alongside overall health. Consulting with a paediatric nutritionist or doctor can help tailor dietary guidelines specific to your unique circumstances.

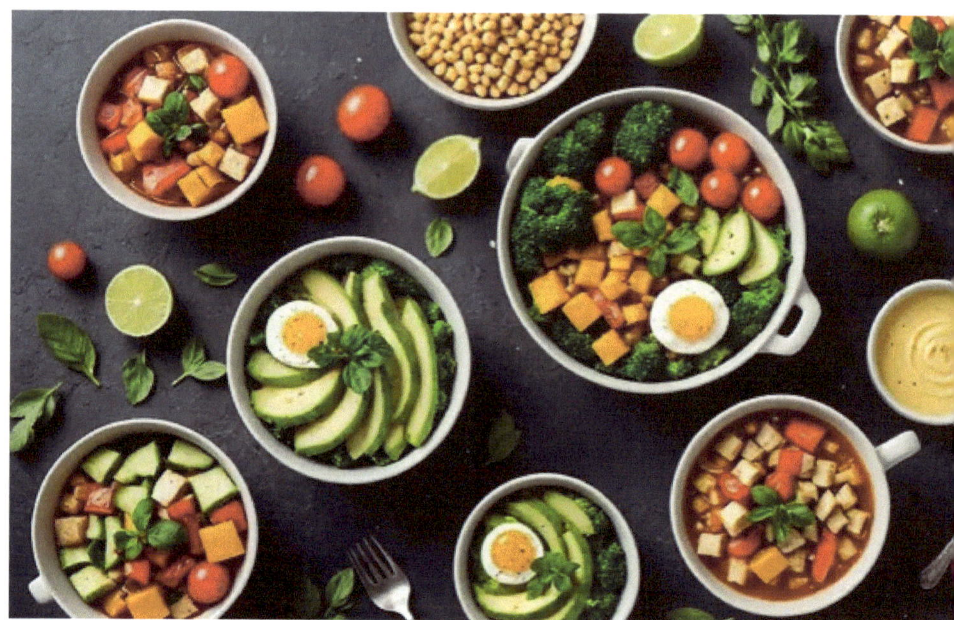

By making informed and healthy choices, you can lay a solid foundation for your baby's future health and development. A well-balanced diet featuring diverse protein sources will benefit both you and your child, ensuring a joyful and nutritious parenting journey.

Chapter 3: Foods to Avoid During Pregnancy

Pregnancy is a wonderful journey, filled with hope and excitement. However, it comes with responsibilities, particularly regarding what you eat. A nutritious diet is essential for both the mother's health and the baby's development. While many foods are beneficial, some carry risks that expectant mothers should be aware of. This guide will highlight foods to avoid, like raw or undercooked meats, high-mercury fish, and unpasteurized dairy products, and will provide safe alternatives to help ensure a healthy pregnancy.

Raw or Undercooked Meat

Risks of Infections and Toxoplasmosis

Eating raw or undercooked meat can expose both the mother and baby to serious health risks. These include foodborne illnesses like listeriosis and salmonella. A staggering 25% of all listeriosis cases occur in pregnant women. Additionally, there is a high risk of toxoplasmosis—a parasitic infection that can lead to severe complications such as miscarriage, stillbirth, and long-term developmental problems in newborns.

Safe Handling and Cooking Tips

To safely enjoy meat during pregnancy, consider the following cooking guidelines:

- **Cook Thoroughly**: Ensure all meats are cooked to safe internal temperatures. Ground meats should be at least 160°F (71°C), while poultry must reach 165°F (74°C).

- **Avoid Cross-contamination**: Use separate cutting boards for raw meat and other foods. Always wash your hands, utensils, and surfaces after handling raw meat.

- **Purchase Fresh**: Buy fresh meat from reputable sources. Always check expiration dates and ensure meats are stored at the correct temperatures.

- **Use a Food Thermometer**: This handy tool can help ensure meats are cooked properly, reducing the risk of foodborne illnesses.

By following these best practices, expectant mothers can significantly decrease their risks while still enjoying a variety of meats.

High-Mercury Fish

Mercury's Impact on Foetal Development

Fish is an important part of a healthy diet due to its omega-3 fatty acids, which are vital for a baby's brain development. However, certain fish contain high levels of mercury, which can harm the baby's nervous system. Research indicates that mercury exposure during pregnancy is linked to a 60% increase in the risk of developmental delays in children.

High-Mercury Fish to Avoid

To eliminate these risks, avoid the following high-mercury fish:

- Shark

- Swordfish

- King mackerel

- Tilefish

- Bigeye tuna

- Raw shellfish (like sushi made with high-mercury fish)

These fish accumulate mercury as they grow, making them unsafe options during pregnancy.

Safer Seafood Options

Fortunately, there are many safe seafood choices that are lower in mercury. Pregnant women should consider including:

- Salmon

- Sardines

- Shrimp

- Catfish

- Pollock

- Cod

These lower-mercury options provide necessary protein and nutrients. Pregnant individuals should aim for up to 12 ounces of low-mercury fish per week to help maintain a balanced diet that supports both their health and their baby's growth.

Unpasteurized Dairy Products

Risk of Listeria and Other Bacteria

Unpasteurized dairy products pose risks during pregnancy, primarily because they can contain harmful bacteria, especially listeria. Listeriosis can cause severe complications like miscarriage or severe illness in newborns. Statistics show that pregnant women are 20 times more likely to develop listeriosis than the general population.

Alternatives and Recommendations

To minimize these risks, opt for pasteurized dairy products, which have been treated to eliminate harmful bacteria. Here are some safer choices:

- Choose pasteurized milk, yogurt, and cheeses that are commonly available in grocery stores.

- Avoid soft cheeses like feta, Brie, and Camembert unless they are made from pasteurized milk.

- Be cautious with deli meats and cold cuts, which can also carry listeria. Heating these until steaming can further reduce the risk.

- Unpasteurized juices should be avoided due to potential harmful bacteria.

The key to a healthy pregnancy is making informed dietary choices. Always read labels and be aware of what you consume to ensure that you and your baby are safe.

Final Thoughts

Nutrition plays a crucial role in ensuring both maternal and foetal health during pregnancy. Avoiding high-risk foods like raw or undercooked meat, high-mercury fish, and unpasteurized dairy products is vital to minimizing health risks. Expectant mothers should prioritize safe food handling practices and choose alternatives that promote wellness.

By making informed choices, new mothers can enjoy a healthy diet while protecting their little ones from potential risks. Always consult healthcare professionals for personalized dietary recommendations throughout your pregnancy journey.

Chapter 4: Managing Pregnancy Cravings and Aversions

Pregnancy is a journey filled with exciting changes, and cravings can spring up unexpectedly. Many expectant mothers find themselves longing for specific foods, while others may suddenly find their favourite meals unappealing. These cravings and aversions are often driven by hormonal shifts and nutritional needs. Understanding how to satisfy these cravings wisely can significantly impact both maternal health and foetal growth. In this guide, we will explore practical swaps for common cravings, provide delicious recipes, and share tips for managing food aversions.

Understanding Pregnancy Cravings

Cravings during pregnancy can vary greatly, ranging from intense desires for sweet treats to aversions to foods that were once enjoyable. Studies indicate that about 50 to 90 percent of pregnant women experience cravings, often for sweet, salty, or high-fat foods. The reasons behind these cravings can involve hormonal changes, nutrient deficiencies, or emotional needs, making it essential to navigate this culinary landscape carefully.

For example, a study published in the "Journal of Nutrition" found that about 85% of women reported craving sweets. Yet, indulging consistently in high-sugar foods may lead to excessive weight gain, potentially impacting pregnancy health.

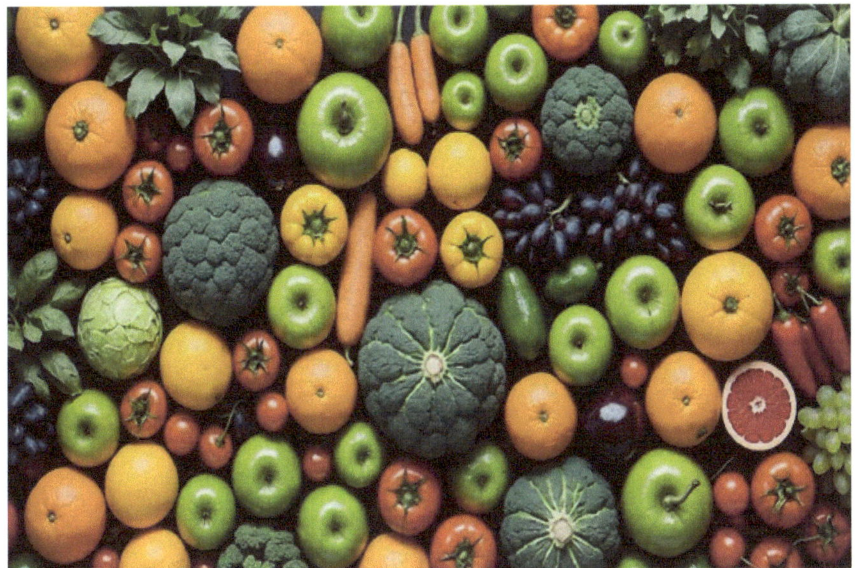

Food aversions can also complicate meal planning, often triggered by increased sensitivity to smells or nausea. Many women may find themselves avoiding healthy options, leading to potential nutritional gaps. Recognizing and understanding these cravings and aversions is key to ensuring both mother and baby receive adequate nutritional support.

Healthy Swaps for Common Cravings

Finding satisfying alternatives for your cravings can help maintain proper nutrition during pregnancy. Here are some simple strategies to enjoy your favourite flavours while staying health conscious.

Satisfying Your Sweet Tooth

Fruits Over Sugary Snacks:

When a sugar craving hits, reach for nature's candy instead. Fresh fruits like strawberries, blueberries, or apples are loaded with vitamins, antioxidants, and dietary fiber. For instance, a cup of strawberries provides about 50 calories, 3 grams of fiber, and more than 100% of your daily vitamin C needs.

Why not whip up a fruit smoothie? Blend together frozen banana, spinach, and yogurt. The yogurt adds protein and calcium, plus the spinach sneaks in additional nutrients without altering the sweet flavour.

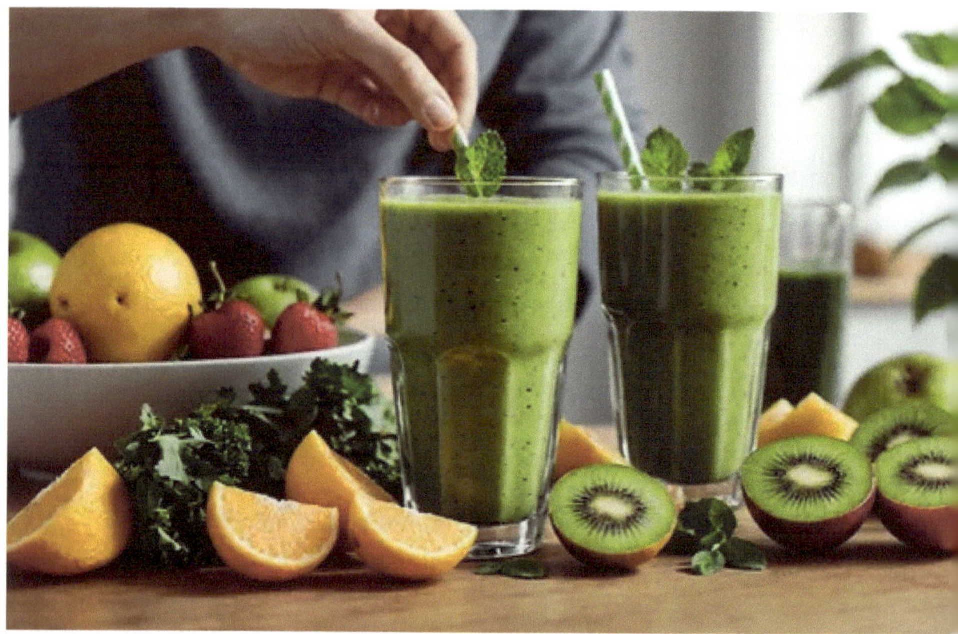

Dark Chocolate:

If you are craving chocolate, choose dark chocolate with 70% cocoa or higher. Dark chocolate is known for its antioxidants, which are beneficial during pregnancy. A 1-ounce serving also offers about 170 calories, providing a guilt-free option to satisfy that sweet tooth. Pair it with a handful of almonds to balance sweetness with healthy fats.

Healthy Baking:

When baking, swap out white flour for whole grain flour or almond flour. This leads to increased fiber and nutrient intake. For example, when making banana muffins, use ripe bananas and oats together, facilitating an easy and nutritious recipe that is perfect for breakfast or snacks.

Addressing Salty Cravings

Nuts and Seeds:

When salt cravings arise, choose unsalted nuts or seeds. A small handful of almonds (about 23 almonds) offers 160 calories, healthy fats, protein, and essential nutrients like vitamin E and magnesium, which are all beneficial during pregnancy.

Air-Popped Popcorn:

Instead of reaching for chips, try air-popped popcorn. This whole grain snack is low in calories and high in fiber, making it a great crunchy alternative. A 3-cup serving of air-popped popcorn contains only 90 calories, and adding a sprinkle of nutritional yeast may give it a savory, cheesy flavour without excess calories.

Hummus with Veggies:

An ideal combo for salty cravings is dipping fresh veggies in hummus. Carrots, cucumber, and bell peppers dipped in hummus offer fiber, vitamins, and healthy fats. For additional flavour, try mixing herbs into your hummus or the veggies.

Delicious Recipes for Cravings

Here are two delightful recipes that combine flavour and nutrition, perfect for tackling cravings.

Fruit & Yogurt Parfait

Ingredients:

- 1 cup of low-fat Greek yogurt

- 1 cup of mixed berries (strawberries, blueberries, raspberries)

- 2 tablespoons of low-sugar granola

Instructions:

1. In a glass or bowl, layer half of the yogurt at the bottom.

2. Add half the mixed berries on top of the yogurt.

3. Sprinkle 1 tablespoon of granola over the berries.

4.   Repeat the layers, finishing with a few berries on top.

This parfait packs protein, antioxidants, and fiber, perfect for starting your day on the right foot.

Nutty Energy Bites

Ingredients:

- 1 cup of oats

- ½ cup of nut butter (peanut or almond)

- ¼ cup of honey or maple syrup

- ½ cup of dark chocolate chips

- ¼ cup of chopped nuts or seeds

Instructions:

1.   In a bowl, combine oats, nut butter, honey, dark chocolate chips, and nuts.

2.   Mix until well combined.

3.   Roll the mixture into bite-sized balls.

4.   Refrigerate for about 30 minutes before enjoying.

These energy bites are a convenient and nutrient-rich snack for any time of the day.

Tips for Dealing with Food Aversions

Food aversions can be just as frustrating as cravings. However, there are practical ways to manage them while ensuring you still get the nutrients you need.

Meal Planning

Keep a Food Diary:

Monitor what you eat and track which foods you dislike. This journal can help you discover patterns and make informed meal-planning decisions, focusing on foods that appeal to you.

Nutritious Substitutions:

If meat does not seem appetizing, consider plant-based proteins such as beans, lentils, or eggs for your protein needs. For greens, blending spinach or kale into a fruit smoothie is a great way to get vital nutrients without tasting the greens.

Creative Meal Combinations:

Experiment with cooking methods. If you find raw vegetables unappealing, try roasting them with spices to bring out their flavours. Adding garlic, rosemary, or other herbs can make them more enticing.

Healthy Options When Foods Feel Unfamiliar

Texture Modifications:

If certain textures push you away, adjust how you prepare your food. For instance, steaming veggies rather than eating them raw can soften their bite and enhance palatability while retaining their benefits.

Mindful Eating:

Focus on smaller, frequent meals to appease both cravings and aversions. Mindful eating allows you to appreciate your food and listen to your body's needs.

Herbal Remedies:

Some expectant mothers find tea helpful in soothing nausea. Ginger or peppermint tea can hydrate while providing digestive benefits. Always check with your healthcare professional first to ensure safety.

Embracing Your Unique Journey

Managing pregnancy cravings and aversions is a balancing act, but it is achievable with thoughtful strategies. By making smart swaps for cravings and craftily planning meals, expectant mothers can ensure both nutrition and satisfaction.

Experimenting with flavours, embracing mindful eating, and staying hydrated all contribute to a healthier pregnancy. Every pregnancy is unique and giving yourself grace to explore these changes can lead to an enjoyable and nourishing experience.

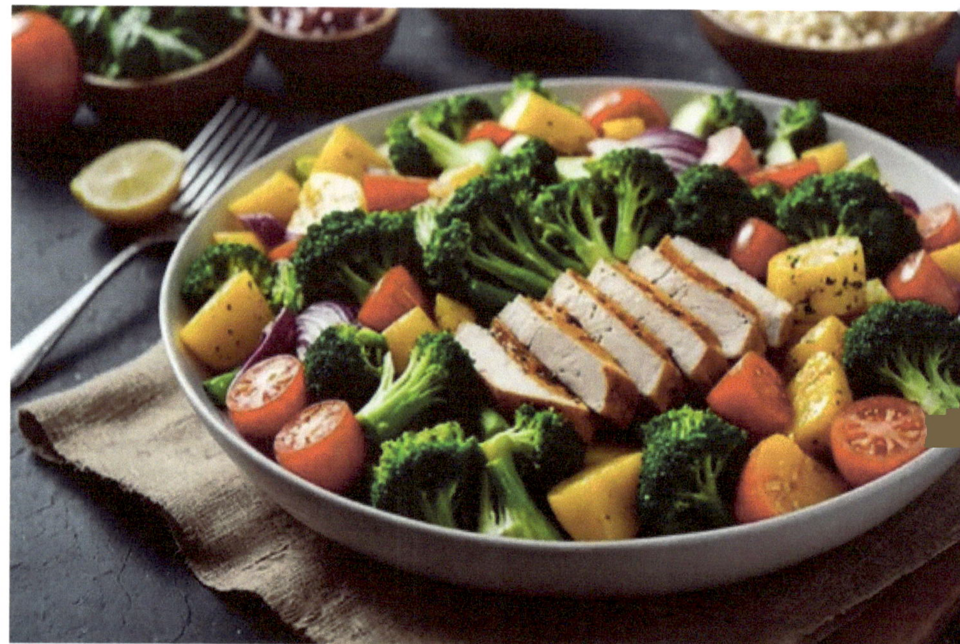

Ultimately, discovering a healthy approach to cravings and aversions makes the journey smoother and helps nurture both you and your growing baby.

Chapter 5: Creating a Balanced Diet Plan for Pregnancy

Pregnancy is an exciting journey, but it also comes with the important task of meeting both the mother's and baby's nutritional needs. A well-balanced diet is crucial during this time, as it supports foetal development, provides energy, and prepares the body for childbirth. In this guide, we will create a nutrient-rich meal plan for pregnancy, including sample daily meal plans, healthy snack ideas, and hydration tips to help you navigate this special time.

Understanding Nutritional Needs in Pregnancy

The nutritional needs of a pregnant woman are different from those of someone who is not pregnant. It is important to focus on nutrient-dense foods that deliver essential vitamins and minerals like:

- **Folic Acid:** Crucial for foetal brain development, found in leafy greens and fortified cereals.

- **Iron:** Supports increased blood volume; red meat, beans, and spinach are good sources.

- **Calcium:** Needed for foetal bone development; dairy products and fortified plant-based milks are excellent choices.

- **Vitamin D:** Supports calcium absorption; consider fatty fish like salmon or fortified milk.

- **Omega-3 Fatty Acids:** Important for brain development, available in fish, walnuts, and flaxseeds.

As pregnancy progresses, caloric needs change. In the first trimester, you may not need additional calories. However, in the second and third trimesters, an increase of about 300-500 calories per day is often necessary. Prioritize these extra calories from nutritious foods rather than empty calories from sugary snacks.

Sample Daily Meal Plans

To simplify meal planning, we have created daily meal plans for each trimester that consider varying nutritional needs and cravings.

First Trimester Meal Plan

In the first trimester, foundational nutrition is crucial. Many women also experience food aversions and nausea, so having easy-to-digest options is key.

Breakfast:

- Whole grain toast topped with half an avocado and a poached egg, providing healthy fats and protein.

- A small bowl of mixed berries, rich in vitamins and antioxidants.

- A glass of fortified orange juice, packed with vitamin C and folic acid.

Morning Snack:

- Greek yogurt drizzled with honey and a sprinkle of cinnamon, supplying calcium and protein.

Lunch:

- Quinoa salad with chickpeas, diced cucumbers, cherry tomatoes, and a lemon-olive oil dressing. Quinoa is a complete protein and can help maintain energy levels.

- A small apple for dessert, delivering fiber and a natural sweetness.

Afternoon Snack:

- Carrot sticks paired with hummus, offering crunch and healthy fats.

Dinner:

- Baked salmon, rich in omega-3 fatty acids, served with steamed asparagus and roasted sweet potatoes.

- A side salad with kale, walnuts, and crumbled feta cheese for added nutrients.

Evening Snack:

- A slice of whole grain toast with almond butter, providing good fats and protein.

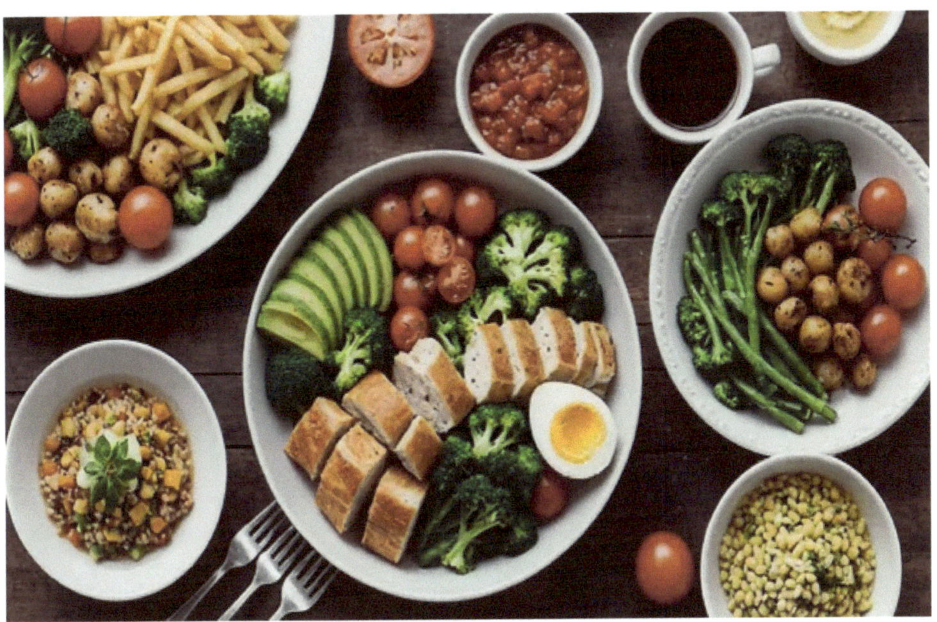

Second Trimester Meal Plan

As the baby grows, the focus shifts to support foetal development and satisfy cravings.

Breakfast:

- A smoothie made with spinach, a banana, Greek yogurt, and almond milk, packed with vitamins and protein.
- A slice of whole grain toast topped with peanut butter, which adds healthy fats.

Morning Snack:

- A small handful of mixed nuts and dried fruits for fiber and energy.

Lunch:

- A turkey and cheese wrap in a whole wheat tortilla, filled with fresh spinach and slices of bell pepper, offering protein and vitamins.
- A side of carrot sticks for extra crunch and nutrition.

Afternoon Snack:

- Whole grain crackers served with guacamole, adding healthy fats and fiber.

Dinner:

- Stir-fried chicken with broccoli and bell peppers, served over brown rice. The chicken is a great protein source, and the veggies offer vitamins and minerals.
- A mixed green salad topped with sliced strawberries and balsamic vinaigrette for additional antioxidants.

Evening Snack:

- Cottage cheese mixed with pineapple chunks for a sweet treat that is high in protein.

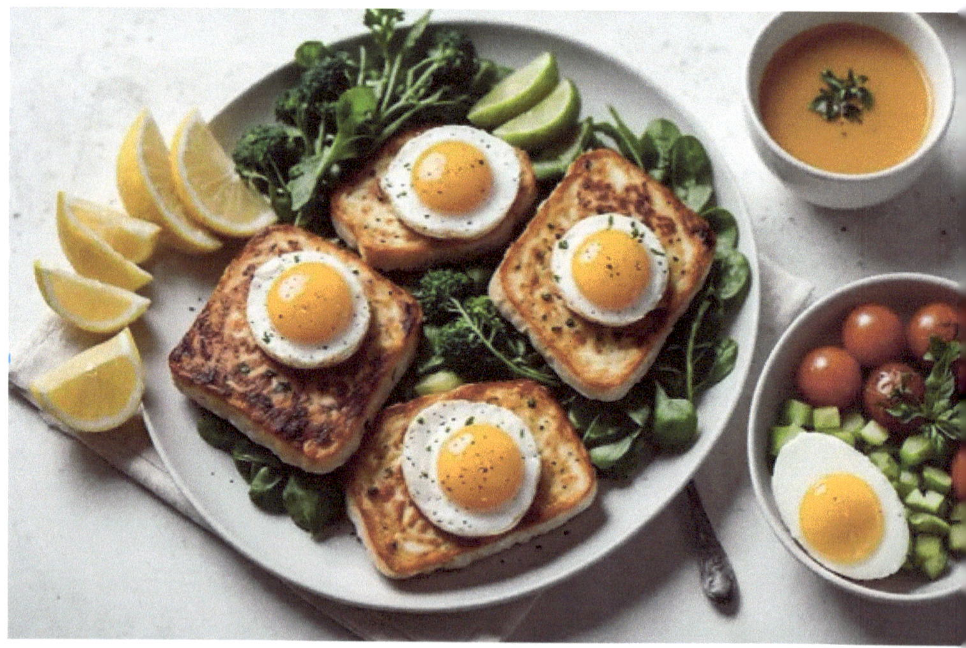

Third Trimester Meal Plan

In the third trimester, meal planning is even more critical due to higher energy needs and the goal of preventing gestational diabetes.

Breakfast:

- Oatmeal topped with fresh fruit, nuts, and a drizzle of honey, providing fiber and steady energy.

- A glass of milk or a milk alternative for calcium.

Morning Snack:

- Sliced apple paired with cheese for a satisfying crunch and protein boost.

Lunch:

- Lentil soup served with whole grain bread, providing fiber and heartiness.
- A side of steamed vegetables for added nutrients.

Afternoon Snack:

- Low-fat yogurt topped with granola for a dose of probiotics and fiber.

Dinner:

- Grilled shrimp tacos with cabbage slaw and avocado in corn tortillas, packed with flavour and healthy fats.
- Quinoa served alongside black beans, offering protein and fiber.

Evening Snack:

- Whole grain muffins loaded with fruit and nuts for a wholesome end to the day.

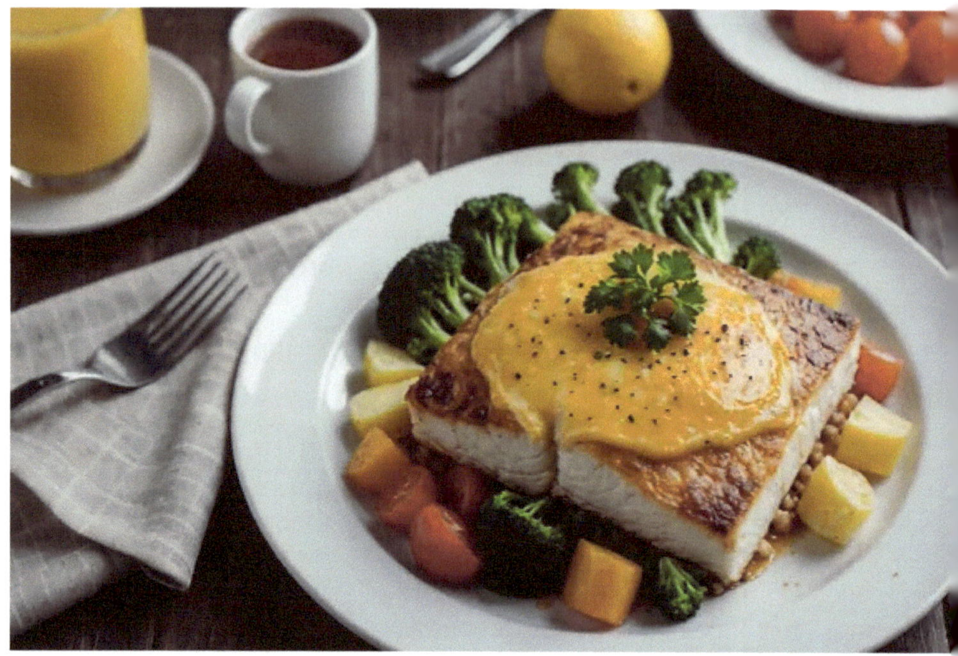

Healthy Snack Ideas

Maintaining steady energy levels is vital during pregnancy. Healthy snacks can help bridge the gaps between meals and keep cravings at bay.

Nutritious Snack Options

- **Fruit and Nut Butter:** Slices of fresh apple or banana paired with almond or peanut butter for a satisfying combination.

- **Yogurt Parfait:** Layer Greek yogurt with granola and fresh fruit for a delicious treat that is high in protein and fiber.

- **Whole Grain Crackers and Cheese:** A simple snack that provides fiber from crackers and protein from cheese.

Easy-to-Make Recipes

1. Energy Bites:

Combine oats, nut butter, honey, and chocolate chips. Roll into small balls and refrigerate for a quick energy snack.

2. DIY Smoothies:

Blend spinach, a banana, yogurt, and a scoop of protein powder for a nutritious smoothie on-the-go.

3. Avocado Toast Variations:

Top whole grain toast with options like sliced tomatoes, a fried egg, or radishes for a tasty treat.

Smart snacking can help satisfy cravings and ensure you are meeting nutritional needs throughout your pregnancy.

Beverages to Consider and Avoid

Staying hydrated is critical during pregnancy. Choosing the right beverages can help you stay hydrated and boost your nutrient intake.

Recommended Beverages

- **Water:** Aim for at least 8-10 cups of water daily to maintain hydration.
- **Herbal Teas:** Enjoy herbal teas like ginger or peppermint for hydration but avoid those that are potentially unsafe.
- **Milk or Milk Alternatives:** Great sources of calcium and vitamin D, supporting bone health.
- **Fresh Juices:** Opt for homemade vegetable juices or 100% fruit juices without added sugars to meet your nutrient needs.

Beverages to Avoid

- **Caffeinated Drinks:** Keep caffeine to a minimum to avoid risks, adhering to recommended guidelines.
- **Alcohol:** The safest approach is complete avoidance, as there is no known safe level during pregnancy.
- **Sugary Soft Drinks:** These can lead to unnecessary weight gain and increase the risk of gestational diabetes.

Focusing on hydration and making thoughtful beverage choices can positively influence your pregnancy.

Wrapping Up

A balanced diet plan during pregnancy is crucial for the health and well-being of both mother and baby. Through careful meal planning with diverse food groups, an emphasis on nutrient-dense options, and smart snacking, mothers can meet their evolving nutritional needs while maintaining energy levels. Be open to adjusting meals and snacks based on cravings and always seek guidance from healthcare professionals regarding nutrition during pregnancy. Enjoy this incredible journey to motherhood!

Chapter 6: Conclusion and Next Steps for a Healthy Pregnancy

Pregnancy marks a significant life event, filled with excitement and joy, but it also brings a lot of responsibilities. For new mothers, ensuring the well-being of both them and their babies is a critical priority. In this post, we will discuss essential aspects of maintaining a healthy pregnancy. We will emphasize the importance of consulting with healthcare professionals, establishing a support plan, and uncovering valuable resources to enhance your journey.

The Importance of Consulting with Healthcare Professionals

Consulting with healthcare professionals during pregnancy is vital for the health and development of both mother and baby.

Regular visits to an obstetrician or midwife provide tailored care and insights that cater to your individual needs. Healthcare providers monitor your health, offer guidance on prenatal care, and create a personalized plan to tackle potential complications. For instance, nearly **2 to 10%** of pregnancies result in gestational diabetes, highlighting the importance of regular check-ups to identify risk factors early.

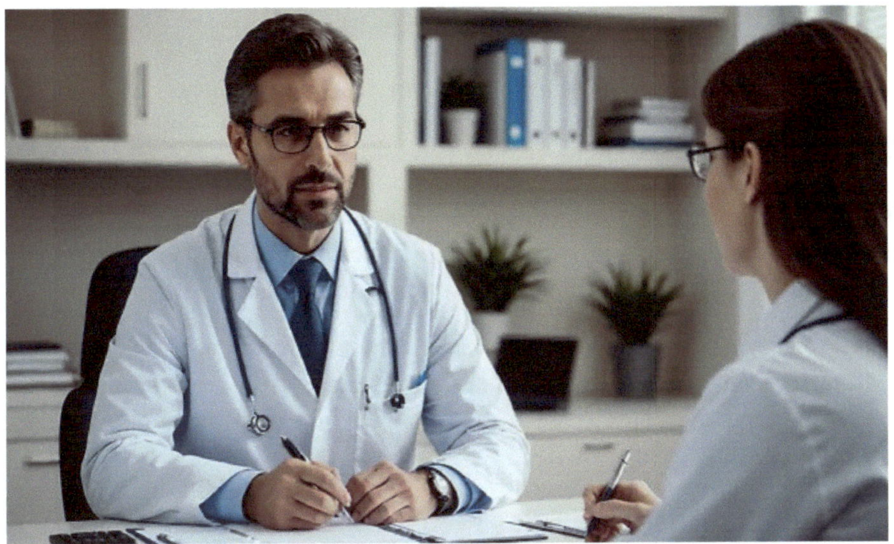

Moreover, routine assessments—such as ultrasounds, blood tests, and genetic screenings—are crucial in tracking foetal development and maternal health. For example, ultrasounds can help identify foetal heart conditions or growth restrictions, which can occur in about **5%** of pregnancies.

In addition to physical health checks, these professionals are instrumental for mental well-being. Pregnancy is often filled with emotional highs and lows. Accessing mental health support from professionals can significantly help manage stress and improve overall wellness.

Establishing Regular Check-Ins with Your Healthcare Provider

Setting up consistent appointments is crucial during your pregnancy. As a guideline, aim for check-ups every four weeks for the first 28 weeks, every two weeks until week 36, and then weekly until delivery. These visits play a pivotal role in ensuring both you and your baby are progressing healthily.

During check-ups, healthcare providers assess various factors, such as weight gain, blood pressure, and foetal heart rates. It is essential to be proactive and discuss any symptoms or concerns you may have.

Creating a Support Plan

A well-structured support system is essential during pregnancy. A support plan includes the people and resources you bring in to navigate this transformative phase without feeling overwhelmed.

Openly communicate your needs with your partner, family, and friends. Discuss how they can support you—be it attending appointments, assisting with household responsibilities, or providing emotional encouragement.

Additionally, consider joining pregnancy support groups, whether local or online. These communities can offer encouragement, share experiences, and provide vital resources, ensuring you feel connected and supported by others on a similar path.

Valuable Resources to Explore

As you embark on the pregnancy journey, utilizing resources will empower you with knowledge and tools vital for a healthy experience. Below, we highlight several guides, websites, and books that you can check out to prepare effectively.

Where to Learn More

1. **Books**: There are many excellent pregnancy books available. One classic recommendation is "What to Expect When You're Expecting," which offers insights into dietary choices, exercise guidelines, and newborn care preparations.

2. **Websites**: Trusted online platforms like the American Pregnancy Association and the Mayo Clinic provide a wealth of helpful information on prenatal care, nutrition advice, weight management, and common pregnancy symptoms.

3. **Pregnancy Apps**: Look for apps that offer features like pregnancy tracking, trimester milestones, and foetal development information. Popular choices like "BabyCenter" and "Ovia Pregnancy" are known for their user-friendly interfaces and rich content.

4. **Birthing Classes**: Enrolling in birthing classes is a great way to prepare for delivery. These classes cover labour and delivery processes, pain management techniques, and newborn care. You

can find local options or choose online classes that fit your preferences.

5. **Prenatal Yoga**: Engaging in prenatal yoga can enhance your physical comfort and mental relaxation. Certified instructors can guide you through safe exercises tailored for expecting mothers.

6. **Consultants and Specialists**: Consider including a lactation consultant, doula, or paediatrician in your care team. These professionals give targeted advice on breastfeeding, childcare preparation, and mental health support.

7. **Hospital Tours**: Scheduling a tour of your delivery hospital can help ease anxiety and familiarize you with the environment. Many hospitals offer informative sessions covering postpartum care and newborn safety practices.

Mental Health Support and Self-Care Techniques

Prioritize your mental well-being by implementing self-care routines during pregnancy. Taking time for yourself can significantly help manage stress. Include activities you enjoy, such as reading, gardening, or spending time in nature.

Make sleep and hydration a priority. These simple practices can improve your mood and energy levels. Incorporating relaxation techniques like deep breathing, meditation, or mindfulness can also help you cope with pregnancy-related anxiety.

Embracing the Journey

Navigating the complexities of pregnancy can be overwhelming at times. However, with the right tools, knowledge, and support, you can thrive during this transformative period.

Consulting healthcare professionals is a cornerstone of healthy pregnancy. They provide personalized care and reassurance, while regular check-ups help address concerns and ensure both you and your baby remain healthy.

Creating a supportive plan and utilizing available resources empower you throughout your pregnancy experience. Whether it is attending prenatal classes, reading informative books, or connecting with supportive communities, every action contributes to a nurturing environment for you and your developing baby.

As you continue on this journey, remember that each pregnancy is unique. Tailor information and recommendations to fit your personal circumstances. Always consult healthcare professionals when making dietary changes or navigating uncertainties.

Empower yourself with knowledge and support and approach the remarkable journey of motherhood with confidence.